This Notebook Belongs To

. . . .

What to Eat

WEEK

	Breakfast	Lunch	Dinner
SUN			
MON			
TUES			
WED			
THURS			
FRI			
SAT			

GROCERY LIST

Notes

Notes

What to Eat

WEEK

	Breakfast	Lunch	Dinner
SUN			
MON			
TUES			
WED			
THURS			
FRI			
SAT			

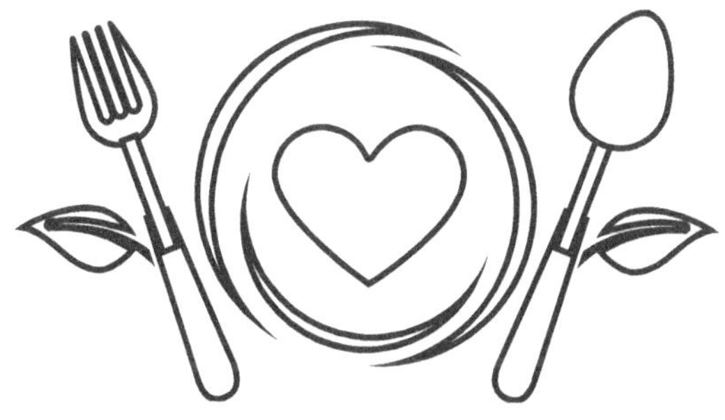

GROCERY LIST

Notes

Notes

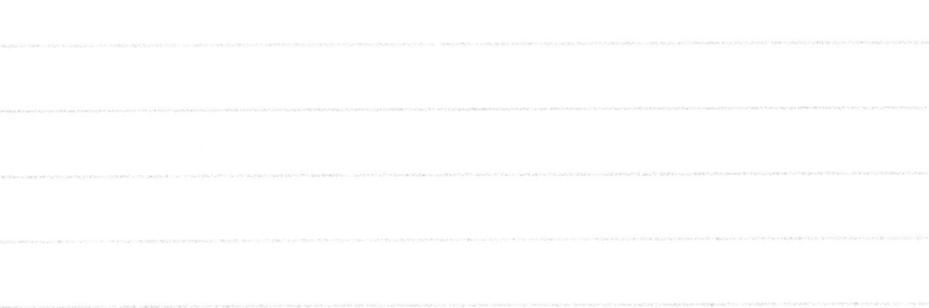

What to Eat

	Breakfast	Lunch	Dinner
SUN			
MON			
TUES			
WED			
THURS			
FRI			
SAT			

GROCERY LIST

Notes

Notes

What to Eat

WEEK

	Breakfast	Lunch	Dinner
SUN			
MON			
TUES			
WED			
THURS			
FRI			
SAT			

GROCERY LIST

Notes

Notes

What to Eat

WEEK

	Breakfast	Lunch	Dinner
SUN			
MON			
TUES			
WED			
THURS			
FRI			
SAT			

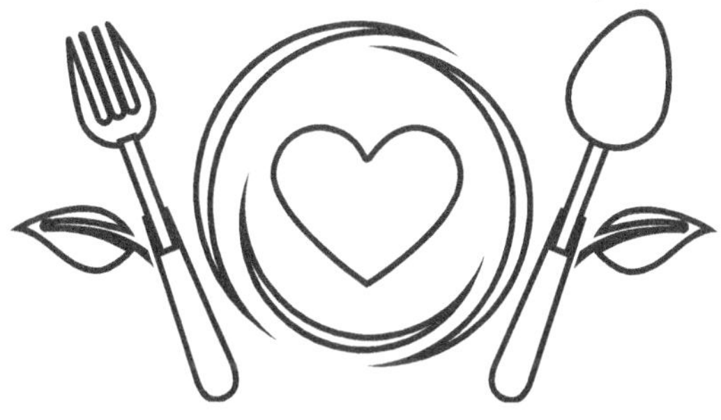

GROCERY LIST

Notes

Notes

What to Eat

WEEK

	Breakfast	Lunch	Dinner
SUN			
MON			
TUES			
WED			
THURS			
FRI			
SAT			

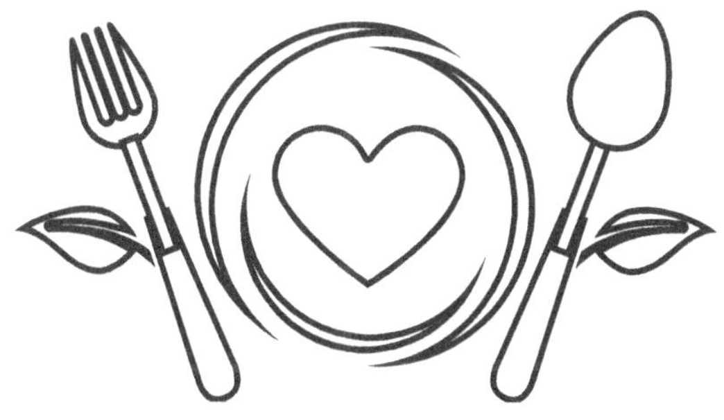

GROCERY LIST

Notes

Notes

What to Eat

WEEK

	Breakfast	Lunch	Dinner
SUN			
MON			
TUES			
WED			
THURS			
FRI			
SAT			

GROCERY LIST

Notes

Notes

What to Eat

WEEK

	Breakfast	Lunch	Dinner
SUN			
MON			
TUES			
WED			
THURS			
FRI			
SAT			

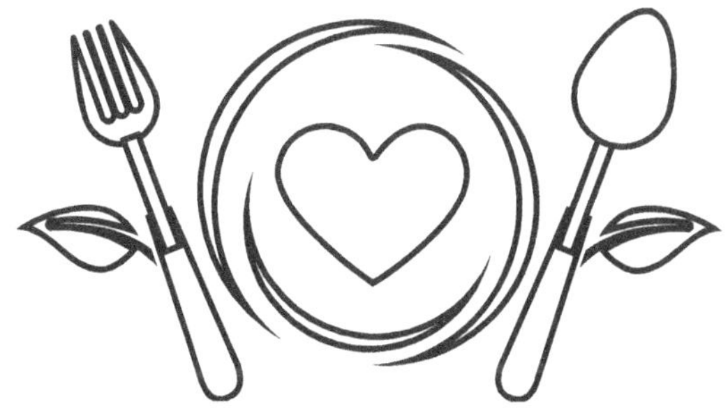

GROCERY LIST

Notes

Notes

What to Eat

WEEK

	Breakfast	Lunch	Dinner
SUN			
MON			
TUES			
WED			
THURS			
FRI			
SAT			

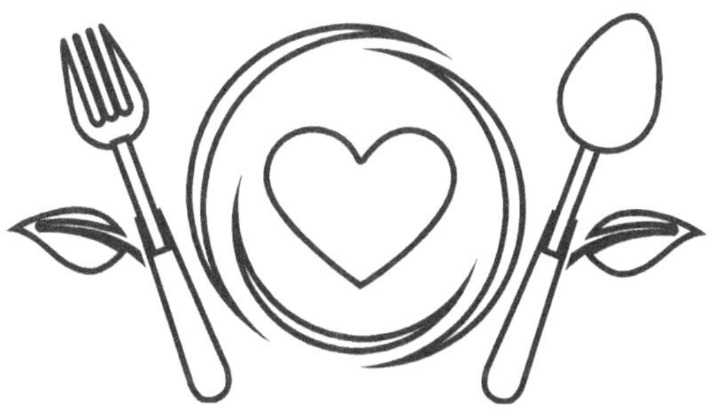

GROCERY LIST

Notes

Notes

What to Eat

WEEK

	Breakfast	Lunch	Dinner
SUN			
MON			
TUES			
WED			
THURS			
FRI			
SAT			

GROCERY LIST

Notes

Notes

What to Eat

WEEK

	Breakfast	Lunch	Dinner
SUN			
MON			
TUES			
WED			
THURS			
FRI			
SAT			

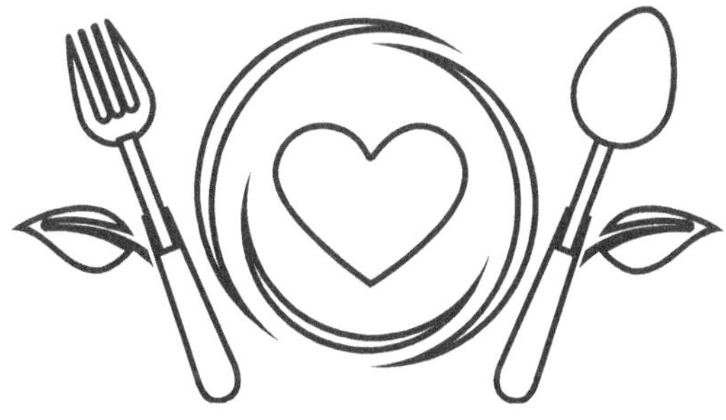

GROCERY LIST

Notes

Notes

What to Eat

WEEK

	Breakfast	Lunch	Dinner
SUN			
MON			
TUES			
WED			
THURS			
FRI			
SAT			

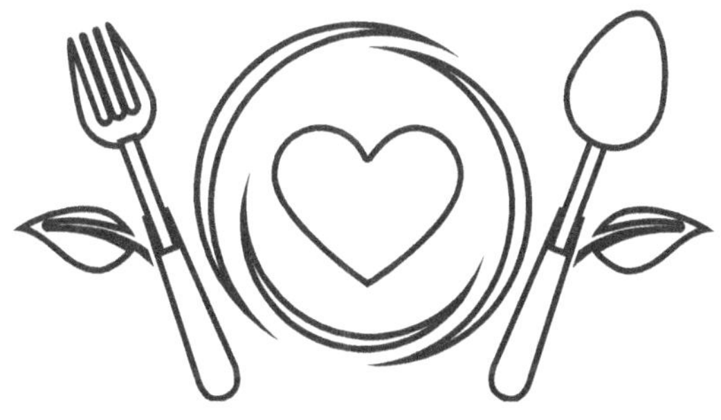

GROCERY LIST

Notes

Notes

What to Eat

WEEK

	Breakfast	Lunch	Dinner
SUN			
MON			
TUES			
WED			
THURS			
FRI			
SAT			

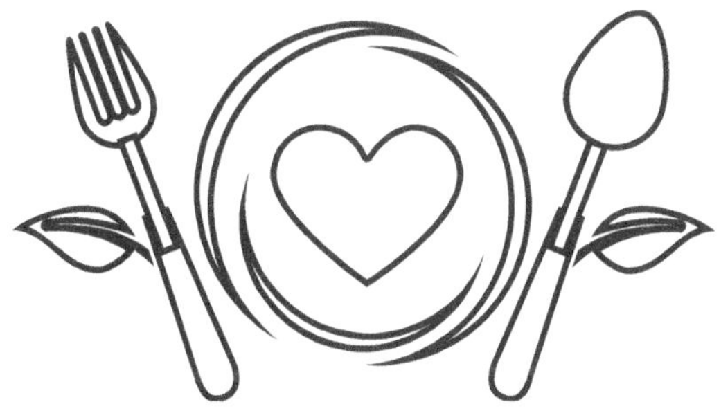

GROCERY LIST

Notes

Notes

What to Eat

WEEK

	Breakfast	Lunch	Dinner
SUN			
MON			
TUES			
WED			
THURS			
FRI			
SAT			

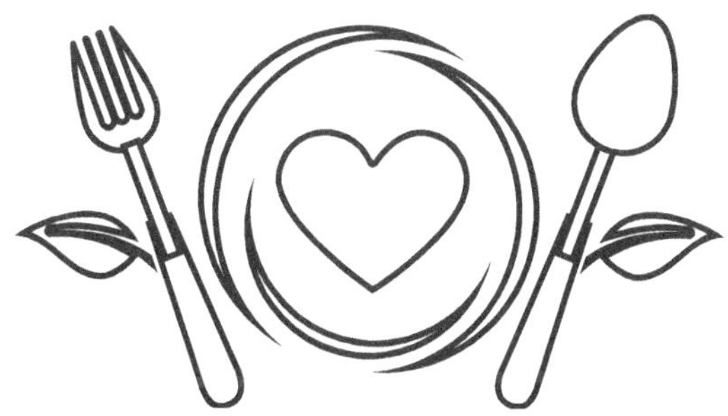

GROCERY LIST

Notes

Notes

What to Eat

	Breakfast	Lunch	Dinner
SUN			
MON			
TUES			
WED			
THURS			
FRI			
SAT			

GROCERY LIST

Notes

Notes

What to Eat

WEEK

	Breakfast	Lunch	Dinner
SUN			
MON			
TUES			
WED			
THURS			
FRI			
SAT			

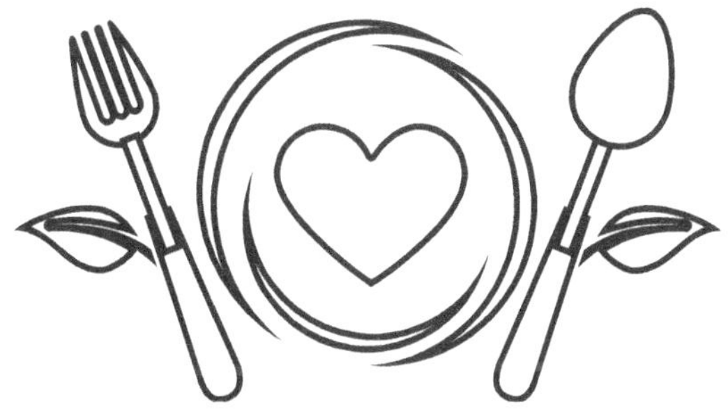

GROCERY LIST

Notes

Notes

What to Eat

WEEK

	Breakfast	Lunch	Dinner
SUN			
MON			
TUES			
WED			
THURS			
FRI			
SAT			

GROCERY LIST

Notes

Notes

What to Eat

WEEK

	Breakfast	Lunch	Dinner
SUN			
MON			
TUES			
WED			
THURS			
FRI			
SAT			

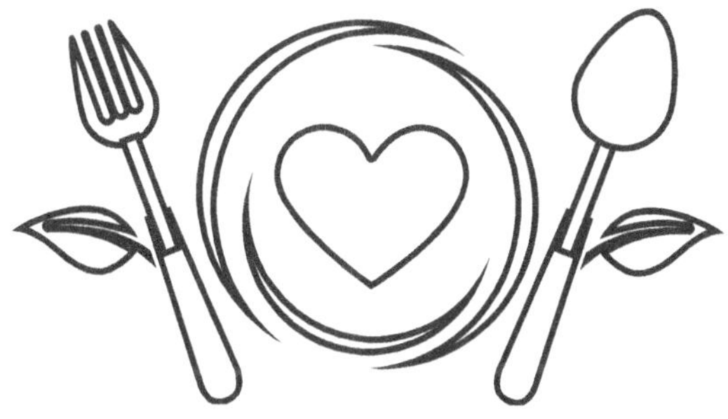

GROCERY LIST

Notes

Notes

What to Eat

	Breakfast	Lunch	Dinner
SUN			
MON			
TUES			
WED			
THURS			
FRI			
SAT			

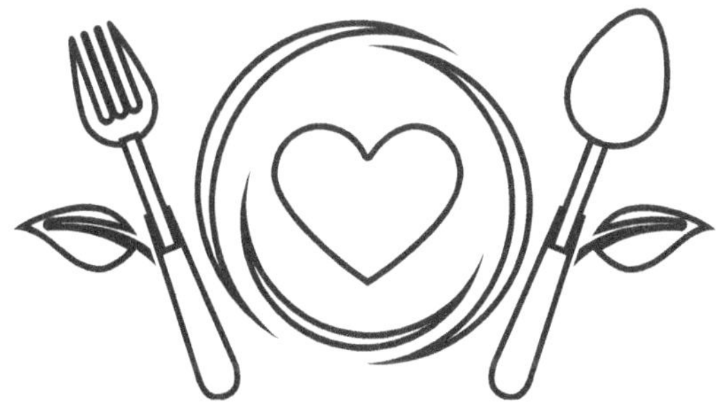

GROCERY LIST

Notes

Notes

What to Eat

WEEK

	Breakfast	Lunch	Dinner
SUN			
MON			
TUES			
WED			
THURS			
FRI			
SAT			

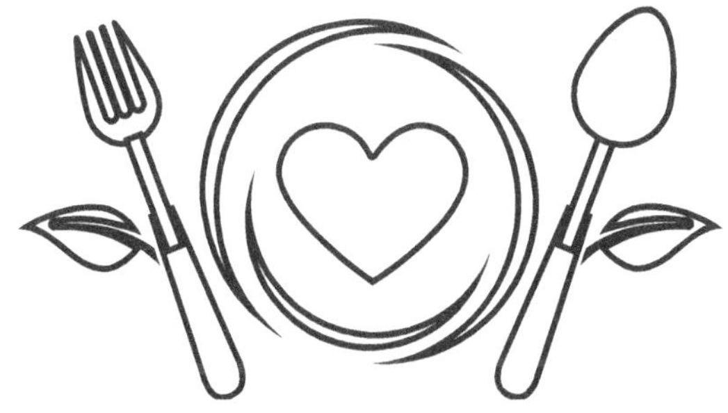

GROCERY LIST

Notes

Notes

What to Eat

	Breakfast	Lunch	Dinner
SUN			
MON			
TUES			
WED			
THURS			
FRI			
SAT			

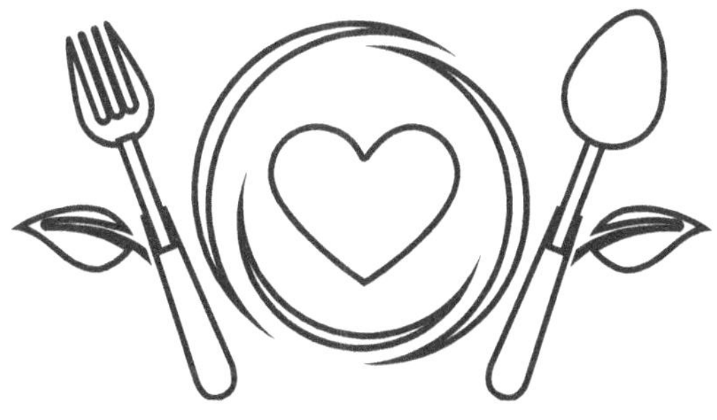

GROCERY LIST

Notes

Notes

What to Eat

WEEK

	Breakfast	Lunch	Dinner
SUN			
MON			
TUES			
WED			
THURS			
FRI			
SAT			

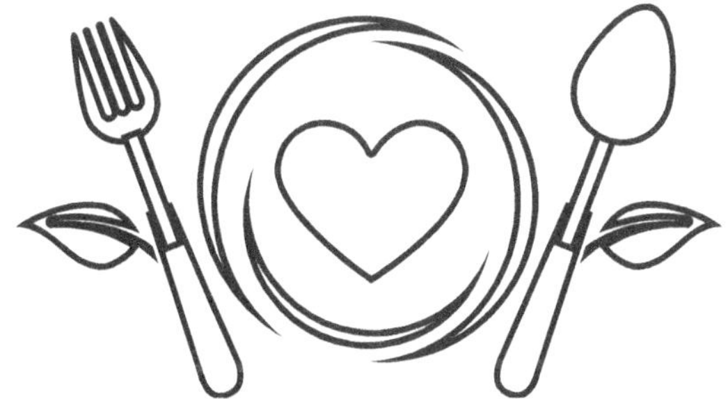

GROCERY LIST

Notes

Notes

What to Eat

WEEK

	Breakfast	Lunch	Dinner
SUN			
MON			
TUES			
WED			
THURS			
FRI			
SAT			

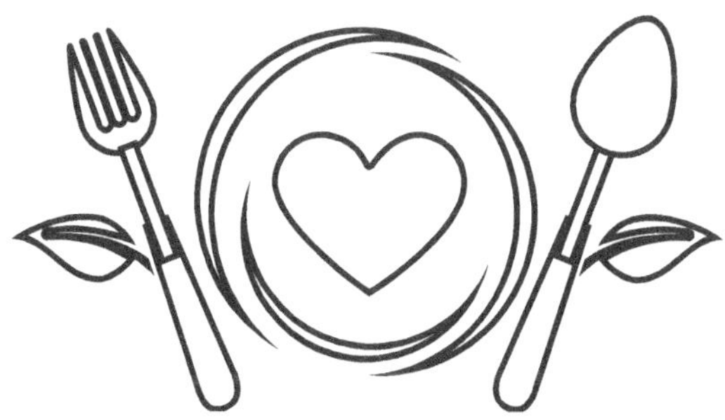

GROCERY LIST

Notes

Notes

What to Eat

WEEK

	Breakfast	Lunch	Dinner
SUN			
MON			
TUES			
WED			
THURS			
FRI			
SAT			

GROCERY LIST

Notes

Notes

What to Eat

WEEK

	Breakfast	Lunch	Dinner
SUN			
MON			
TUES			
WED			
THURS			
FRI			
SAT			

GROCERY LIST

Notes

Notes

What to Eat

WEEK

	Breakfast	Lunch	Dinner
SUN			
MON			
TUES			
WED			
THURS			
FRI			
SAT			

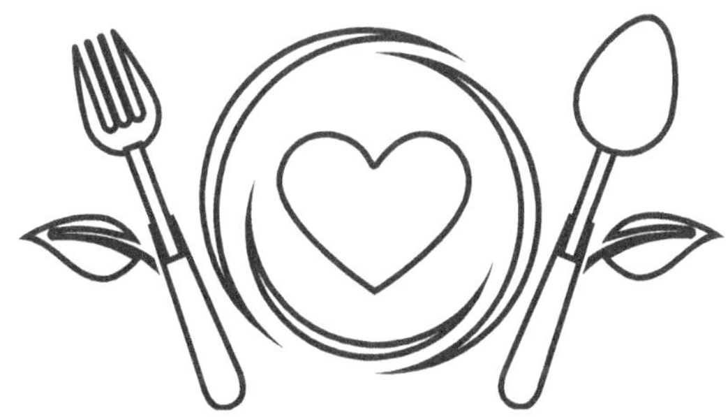

GROCERY LIST

Notes

Notes

Notes

THANK YOU!

LET US KNOW HOW YOU LIKE OUR NOTEBOOK AT:

G.PUBLISHING.E@GMAIL.COM